WITH A
COMES HOPE
VOLUME ONE

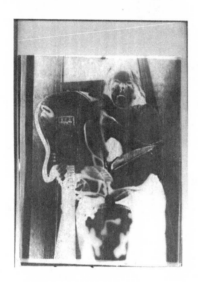

By Helen Care

'One million people commit suicide every year'
The World Health Organization

Helen Care

Published by
Chipmunkapublishing
PO Box 6872
Brentwood
Essex CM13 1ZT
United Kingdom

http://www.chipmunkapublishing.com

Edited by Shareen Ali

"With Anger Comes Hope"

Volume One

By

Helen Care

June 2007

Helen Care

WITH ANGER COMES HOPE

This book is dedicated to the

Memory of my grandfather

Norman Bentley

1911 – 2007

"No person is ever truly alone.

Those who live no more,

Whom we loved,

Echo still within our thoughts.

Our words, our hearts

And what they did and who they were

Become a part of all that we are

Forever"

Helen Care

WITH ANGER COMES HOPE

I have been a Mental Health Service User for almost thirteen years now and only recently returned to work as a Mental Health Outreach Support Worker.

For as long as I can remember, I have been troubled by my life's events and found an escape in the form of poetry. I started writing poems in my early teens and have never stopped. I found this creative process an ongoing cathartic tool in restoring my mental wellbeing.

I am also a singer/song writer, playing the guitar and keyboards. I used to be in a band called "Procyclidine!!" which was great fun! Something to return to and explore in the future? Maybe.

I believe I am back on track!

Helen Care

ANGER

Anger spinning round
Anger in my brain
Anger deep inside
Makes me feel the pain

Anger from the hurt
Anger from the past
Anger from the present
For anger seems to last

Time to face the anger
Time to learn to cope
Time to stop the cutting
Time to see the hope

September 1996

Helen Care

Got It Sussed

Back on track
For I lost my way
In the wilderness
I hear you say

Feeling calm
At long last
I can smile now
I can laugh….so I'll…

Take my time
To readjust
The worst is over
I've got it sussed

Anxiety's gone
I feel positive
Looking forward
No longer negative

I can remember
How I felt
Lost and scared
The cards were dealt….so I'll…

Take my time
To readjust
The worst is over
I've got it sussed

But I can determine

WITH ANGER COMES HOPE

My own destiny
I can take control
And live in reality

For there is hope
I won't live to die
I've woken up
I won't cry….but I'll…

Take my time
To readjust
The worst is over
I've got it sussed

December 2005-February 2006

Helen Care

Charmed And Chilled

White grinning teeth
Does happiness lie beneath?
Pink smiling lips
Do you want to quit?

Quit while you're ahead
Doing headstands on your head
Bouncing around the fire
Time to stop being such a liar

So charmed and chilled
Is this something instilled?
Inside you trying to get out
Do you want to scream and shout?

Liar, liar – such fantasies
No such chilled memories
Thoughts erased and left
For you to save and fetch

Fetch up your white teeth
Does happiness lie beneath?
Pink smiling lips
Do you want to quit?

So charmed and chilled
Is this something instilled?
Inside you trying to get out
Do you want to scream and shout?

May 2006

12

WITH ANGER COMES HOPE

ADRENALIN RUSH

Life can be stressful
With what you're doing
Try not to get wasted
It's only you, you're fooling

Maybe in the midst
Of your mid-life crisis
Your hatred for hangovers
Leads you to psychosis

Perpetuate an image
Without the pitfalls
Need to explain time
Without growing tall

There on the roadside
A moment in time
A hitchhiker in love
Searching for a sign

In such moments of beauty
Creating such euphoria
Life's hanging around
Incredulous hysteria

Sitting here damaged
What's the substance?
A nervous disposition
Of such decadence

Mental stimulation

Helen Care

Intellectual realisation
Silenced to a hush
For your adrenalin rush

<u>January 2005</u>

WITH ANGER COMES HOPE

DYING TO LIVE

You were born at the crack of dawn
A restless child sometimes wild
You made such a noise broke your toys
Went to school and broke every rule

What they called teaching you called
preaching
Between your jests they dealt out tests
But you never worked always shirked
You should've looked out but got chucked out

When you lost your aim, they forgot your name
Just one of the three million riding pillion
It was through the town you got tied down
She had the baby someone else's maybe

Your very own child growing up wild
Wouldn't learn so started to earn
Began to spend but soon to lend
Skipped on tax forgetting the facts

Lost your job becoming one of the mob
You took to drinking stopped your thinking
Had too much leisure and little pleasure
Soon fell ill and lost your will

Developed senility ending in fatality
Died in peace ending the lease
No one around to shed a tear
Like there was no-one dear
<u>1983/2001</u>

Comforting Tonight

A flash of inspiration
A flash of white light
A flash of realisation
It's comforting tonight

To know I'm okay
To know I'm not evil
To know I'm not in the wrong
This has been such an upheaval

It's okay to have a different view
It's okay to believe you're not wrong
This does not make me evil
But why has it taken so long?

Years of pressure and fear
Years of God, Bad and Evil
Reached a point of no return
I've escaped Hell – but will I burn?

A flash of inspiration
A flash of white light
A flash of realisation
It's comforting tonight

March 2002

WITH ANGER COMES HOPE

Love Is What You Bring

You start to laugh
Tugging at my strings
That adorns my heart
Love is what you bring

Shoot a withering look
As you grab at my wrist
Don't want to be let down
Trust me and take a risk

I've got your jumper
Do you want it back?
For it's kept me warm
So cut me some flack

Chat away amiably
Bright – eyed and clear
Never a cross moment
Love you hold so dear

Share all your secrets
That darkens your heart
Step out into the open
Feel the chains fall apart

We've plenty in common
We have the same past
The present is where we're at
Will our future last?

Helen Care

You start to laugh
Tugging at my strings
That adorns my heart
Love is what you bring

December 2005

WITH ANGER COMES HOPE

Is This A Dream?

Please hold me in your arms
Protect me from all harm
Seal your love with a kiss
And grant my only wish

To be yours for all time
Soul mates so always kind
Tender to all my needs
Don't break up, darling please

I thought I heard a scream
Am I asleep?
I thought it was me
Is this a dream?

Move closer with your love
Blessed from Heaven above
Feeling safe in my sleep
And from my waking dream

I know I toss and turn
Support me with concern
Hug me with your embrace
Life with you I can face

I thought I heard a scream
Am I asleep?
I thought it was me
Is this a dream?

October 2004

Helen Care

A Magical Cure

I want what I can't have
I want my life back
I want to be a child again
But with a different ending

But will it make me happy?
Will it make me feel secure?
Is there a fairytale ending?
I wish there was a magical cure

I want what I lost out on
I want love without burden
I want to be happy again
And laugh without any shame

I want what I dreamed of
I want to be able to rise above
I want to be untouched
And clean for I've had enough

I want what I'm owed
I want an apology and honesty
I want to be believed
And guilt for you to concede

But will it make me happy?
Will it make me feel secure?
Is there a fairytale ending?
I wish there was a magical cure

2003

WITH ANGER COMES HOPE

<u>Middle Ground</u>

All that guilt
All that blame
All that hurt
Feeling full of shame

Violence and hate
Help came too late
The legacy lives on
Anger's already begun

All that fear
All that sex
All that love
Fearful of what next

Violence and hate
Help came too late
The legacy lives on
Anger's already begun

All those stories
All those lies
All those words
Feelings I can't hide

Violence and hate
Help came too late
The legacy lives on
Anger's already begun

All that jazz

Helen Care

All that cover-up
All that deceit
Feeling so incomplete

Trying to find a middle ground
Let go of feelings that abound
Trying to find a middle ground
My heart was never found

<u>February 2003</u>

WITH ANGER COMES HOPE

WEAPONS OF MASS DESTRUCTION

Convinced us into war
What were we fighting for?
Like so many times before
Your decisions have left us raw

Fuelled by oil and greed
Did you think that we'd concede?
Made a stand and took the lead
Not happy until we bleed

A loss of innocent lives
Their future so deprived
Western hype and selfish lies
There is no place for you to hide

We're now reeling the costs
Your explanation is at such a loss
You won't convince us because
You're full of shit-we've had enough

Now sat here and upon reflection
We're sick and tired of your projection
That we should greet your suggestion
Conquering the enemy's infection

Weapons of Mass Destruction
In isolation
Such alienation
Weapons of Mass Destruction

January 2004

Helen Care

HORRIFIED

Such horrifying footage
Of prisoners being abused
A hooded captive on a box
Wires attached and ready to fuse

Naked and stacked in a
Human pyramid – jeered
So inhumanely by soldiers
Laughing almost in fear

If you fall off the box
You will be electrocuted
Pose in humiliating stands
Simulating acts so polluted

The captive "Broke within hours"
For there is no excuse for this
So appalled and concerned
At such a display we can't dismiss

Orders of many beatings
In an attempt for them to talk
Were they just following orders?
Or is it they've now been caught?

Are these distressing images
Too much for us to live with?
What happened to dignity and respect?
Is this something we can forgive?

If you fall off the box

24

WITH ANGER COMES HOPE

You will be electrocuted
Pose in humiliating stands
Simulating acts so polluted

<u>June 2004</u>

Panic

Do you have the one last drink?
When you know it will make you sick
Do you smoke just one more joint?
Good or bad – what's your point?

Do you sleep with the only guy?
That's spent all night chatting you up
Do you try and 'chase the dragon'?
When you know what you will become

When I'm cold inside
Please make me feel warm
When I'm frightened
Please hold my hand
When I'm in distress
Please make me feel safe
When I'm feeling destructive
Please take away the blade

Do you think it's time to give up?
On life that passes you by
Motivation is slow
How low do you go?

Red stands for the panic button
All that pain that I'd forgotten
Has come back to haunt me
The place I'm in is worse than reality

When I'm cold inside
Please make me feel warm

26

WITH ANGER COMES HOPE

When I'm frightened
Please hold my hand
When I'm in distress
Please make me feel safe
When I'm feeling destructive
Please take away the blade

February 2004

Helen Care

As A Child

As a child
I had an ability
To retain
Your difficulty

As a child
I miraculously
Coped with
Your insanity

As a child
I was planted
With your seed
Then taken for granted

As a child
My generosity
You exploited
So demandingly

As a child I lent
You my trust
Which you abused
For your own lust

As a child I thought
You'd disappear
If I was to tell
This was such a fear

As a child I was

WITH ANGER COMES HOPE

So frightened
My sensitivity
Was so heightened

**As a child
My generosity
You exploited
So demandingly**

<u>November 2004</u>

The Truth Can't Be Fixed

So many boys and girls
Armed only with stones
Taunt unfriendly soldiers
Who retaliate with undertones?

What starts as a game
Ends up in terror
Shot at and arrested
Crimes so hard to measure

As the sun rises
Over the horizon
It's already starting
To heat up the division

Your pounding heart
And sweaty brow
Have little to do with
The rising sun right now

As you climb out
Of your overwhelming fear
Trapped in the barbed wire
You start to shed a tear

Travel to the checkpoint
Have a rifle in your face
Left to stand in the blazing sun
You can't escape this place

Arrested on your way home

WITH ANGER COMES HOPE

Accused of imaginary crimes
Denied access to information
As to whether you survived

Children put on trial
Scapegoats in politics
So corrupt and unjust
The truth can't be fixed

May 2007

Helen Care

<u>SO</u>

The power to see
The power to speak
A continuum
So please
Watch yourself
Like a child
Needs love
So try.

Nothing is familiar
So lost in a world
Of lifeless ambitions
So swirl
Such a visual world
Speak about things
Face to face
So understanding.

**Fits like a glove
On your hand
It's so snug
So unplanned**

<u>**February 2005**</u>

WITH ANGER COMES HOPE

Ease Her Fears

He had a strong smile
Complete with shiny teeth
He closed his eyes for a while
Remembering his belief...

That greeted her with tenderness
Assuming her need for comfort
He opened his arms to confess
His love for her and all her hurt...

That she carried in her heart
Waiting to be loved and consoled
In a world so battered and stark
It's time to look after your soul

A painful tension
She always felt
But forgot to mention
To anyone else

Moving with deliberate gestures
That is implanted in your mind
With a sense of perfect measures
That lives up to your love so blind

In trust she flowed out to him
She's feeling grateful and warm
As he has a special place, that's in
Her heart that shines at dawn

For he has harmonious manners

Helen Care

That is never sudden or violent
She feels threatened by daggers
Revealed when she was silent

A painful tension
She always felt
But forgot to mention
To anyone else

Now she's tired by his energy
That only serves to wear her out
She's not as young unfortunately
As she feels so full of doubt

She loves his caressing voice
That reassures her love for him
She feels that he gives her a choice
To reach a place they can't begin

To be in tune with each other
Giving room for understanding
To love and grow together
Where life isn't demanding

Her painful tension
Has now disappeared
He has remembered
To ease her fears

February 2006

WITH ANGER COMES HOPE

<u>Being Blamed</u>

Walking away
From a part of me
Change direction
Find a street

To escape from
Being alone
Take my place
Take me home

While I'm here
I feel guilt
So responsible
Hurt has built

Up like a tower
That stands tall
Climb the steps
Don't you fall?

From a routine
That numbs
My senses
Come undone

**You failed
You rejected
You sustained
Being blamed**

Helen Care

I need shelter
From your storm
In a tea cup
To keep me warm

So you repeat
Every change
To protect me
Every day

Feel my sorrow
Wash your eyes
Cleanse your face
From your lies

Clap your hands
Stamp your feet
Dance the dance
And live your dream

So make a wish
That is true
To your soul
Right on cue

You failed
You rejected
You sustained
Being blamed

February 2006

WITH ANGER COMES HOPE

(I'm) Not At Your Disposal

Repeated trauma
Erodes the structure
Already formed
Now so deformed

Trapped little child
Bursting so wild
Black depression
Task of adaptation

Just leave me alone
I want to be on my own
I've nearly had my full
(I'm) Not at your disposal

Must find a way
Allow me to say
I sense your trust
For me it's just lust

Safety is so unsafe
Control face to face
You're so unpredictable
Yet so spiritual

Trauma of structure
Formed but deformed
A child so wild
Depression of adaptation

Helen Care

A way to say
Trust means lust
Unsafe to face
Unpredictably spiritual

Helplessness
Failure told her
Care if you dare
Senses are my defences

Power of helplessness
Everything's such a mess
Cope with failure
So like, he told her

Failures at care
Hit, only if you dare
Scared of my senses
It's just my defences

Just leave me alone
I want to be on my own
I've nearly had my full
(I'm) Not at your disposal

August 2003

WITH ANGER COMES HOPE

What a Struggle

I don't want to spend the rest of my days
In fear and dread of everything you say
I need to find some peace of mind
Something I doubt I'll ever find

This I'll only achieve when you're dead and gone
Leaving me empty in spite of new found freedom
Why with you, can there be no compromise
All I want is to stop feeling so bad inside

What a struggle I have with my life
He shouldn't have sex with me, but with his wife
All you have done is cause me trouble and strife
What a struggle I have with my life

You're in my dreams and in my nightmares
You're in my flashbacks leaving me so scared
Wish I could tear it all down and start again
I'm very good at playing out your games

But now I've had enough of this hurt
That you've dealt out, treating me like dirt
Well now, it's time for me to be released
So will I forget you ever exist?

What a struggle I have with my life
He shouldn't have sex with me, but with his wife

Helen Care

**All you have done is cause me trouble and
strife
What a struggle I have with my life**

<u>**March 2004**</u>

WITH ANGER COMES HOPE

From This Place

Tear through the streets
With alarming beats
That tears your flesh
Burning you no less

Will your heart burn
If you fall out of turn
The long cry of alarm
Reminds you of harm

You appeared to subside
When invited to climb
Balancing on the ladder
You try not to swagger

You look with a frown
Too scared to look down
It's so hard to sit still
When you chase the thrill

This child survived
From deep inside
This child felt safe
From this place

Breathless with fear
Uncomfortable to hear
The silence of the past
Is it destined to last?

Helen Care

Impatient, yet alert
To all of your hurt
Restless, yet so keen
To your every dream

Your smile's so sweet
Keeps me on my feet
But don't lose your grip
Hold on with your wit

You drift towards the door
This intensity you can't ignore
So you plan your escape
You're ready to leave this place

This child survived
From deep inside
This child felt safe
From this place

February 2006

WITH ANGER COMES HOPE

In Awe of What Next

It's not a surprise to materialise
All your feelings that leave you reeling
Your eyes are watching me scratching
Out a rhythm, am I forgiven?

Breathing deeply
Take long steps
So completely
In awe of what next

So close up together will this last forever?
Just like a child feeling so fragile
You walk in step with me such an assured reality
You glance and smile just once in a while

Breathing deeply
Take long steps
So completely
In awe of what next

And then you vanished as if you were banished
Mirrors have a vain life, which has never been
right
Time to confront yourself don't sink into your shell
Start a walk to the truth stay strong along this
route

Breathing deeply
Take long steps
So completely
In awe of what next

Helen Care

Have a sense of the dangers of those who were
strangers
Such precise moments of power, that thwarted
you at every hour
In a mood of such weakness when there was
much bleakness
My memory is still intact secrets are no longer our
pact

Breathing deeply
Take long steps
So completely
In awe of what next

<u>February 2006</u>

WITH ANGER COMES HOPE

Put It Right

A flush of pleasure
Ran so deep
It's hard to measure
Try to sleep

A glistening smile
Seems so false
Just for a while
Feel my pulse…

That beats so fast
But will it last?
Before I give in
For you to be forgiven….

For every mistake
For all your hate
That dragged me down
Just like your frown…

That filled me with fear
Were you ever sincere?
With your love for me
That should've set me free

Feeling under pressure
With your demands
For my treasure
Is in your hands

Helen Care

I wish I could run
Flee this place
For you have won
This wretched race

So please let me go
To recover you know
But I'm scared to feel
The pain is far too real

For my emotions
Were dampened
So I could function
At every junction

**That needed direction
And a resurrection
To get back my life
And to put it right**

February 2006

WITH ANGER COMES HOPE

RISE AND FALL

IF YOU KNOW SOMEONE WHO IS
STRUGGLING
LEND THEM A HAND TO START PADDLING
OUT OF THE DEEP SEA THAT CAN OVERTAKE
YOU
JUMP OVER THE WAVES THAT'LL ALWAYS
CONTINUE

**SO RISE AND FALL, WAVE BY WAVE
YOU STAND SO TALL, YOU ARE SO BRAVE**

TO FIND THE TRUTH SO VOID OF LIES
TRUTH CAN SET YOU FREE NOW YOU CAN
FLY
WE NEED TO BELIEVE AND TO HAVE HOPE
THAT'LL HELP US GROW, THAT'LL HELP US
COPE

**SO RISE AND FALL, WAVE BY WAVE
YOU STAND SO TALL, YOU ARE SO BRAVE**

UNPLUGGED FROM LIFE FEELING SO
DEFENSELESS
DO YOUR TACTICS LEAVE YOU POWERLESS?
A SPIRITUAL COMMITMENT OR IS THAT JUST
A THEORY?
I'VE GOT LOTS OF QUESTIONS THAT I NEED
TO QUERY

**SO RISE AND FALL, WAVE BY WAVE
YOU STAND SO TALL, YOU ARE SO BRAVE**

PLEASE RESPOND TO MY NEEDS, ANSWER
ALL MY QUESTIONS
THAT ARE SO CHALLENGING I NEED TO
MAKE DECISIONS
WE DON'T HAVE TO PROVE THAT WE ARE
VERY KIND
FOR WE HAVE LOVE WE HAVE PEACE OF
MIND

**SO RISE AND FALL, WAVE BY WAVE
YOU STAND SO TALL, YOU ARE SO BRAVE**

<u>FEBRUARY 2006</u>

WITH ANGER COMES HOPE

TIME TO HEAL

I'M ALWAYS LOOKING
FOR SOMETHING
OUT OF NOTHING

I FEEL SO LOST
AT WHAT COST
MAKE IT STOP

LET ME GO
TAKE IT SLOW
YOU SHOULD KNOW

HOW I SHOULD FEEL
TRY TO KEEP IT REAL
MY LOVE YOU DID STEAL
GIVE ME TIME TO HEAL

START AGAIN
ON THE MEND
DON'T KNOW WHEN

I'LL FEEL LOVED
LIKE GOD ABOVE
I'VE HAD ENOUGH

OF ALL THE SINNERS WHO
THINK THEY'RE WINNERS
JUST BEGINNERS....WHO SHOULD KNOW

HOW I SHOULD FEEL
TRY TO KEEP IT REAL

49

Helen Care

MY LOVE YOU DID STEAL
GIVE ME TIME TO HEAL

YOU SHOULD KNOW
TAKE IT SLOW
LET ME GO

MAKE IT STOP
AT WHAT COST
I FEEL LOST

OUT OF NOTHING
COMES SOMETHING
I'M ALWAYS LOOKING… AS YOU SHOULD
KNOW

HOW I SHOULD FEEL
TRY TO KEEP IT REAL
MY LOVE YOU DID STEAL
GIVE ME TIME TO HEAL

FEBRUARY 2006

WITH ANGER COMES HOPE

A Sense of Calm

Building up to a point
Not really sure where to go
Feeling so overwhelmed
Trying hard not to let it show

So glad of your support
Space to feel at ease
Comfortable to let go
Of all those demons I see

Starting to open my eyes
To all that vulnerability
That accompanied my guilt
It only heightened my sensitivity

Gremlins pop-up unannounced
Frightening me like hallucinations
So scary in everyday life
Can't sleep due to recriminations

Invade my space and mind
Attempting to break my sanity
Do I need to take a step back?
To reflect on your inhumanity

But I will rise up from the floor
With love and support I will grow
Don't want to know you anymore
So detrimental to me you know

Helen Care

A sense of calm **takes over**
Regain my breath and composure
Fight the hate, drugs and alcohol
Try and get a sense of closure

You're so good for my mental health
Talk, think and take a breath
To consider my fearfulness
At events and feelings I confess

October 2003

WITH ANGER COMES HOPE

DO YOU SEE ME LAUGHING?

SO OVERWHELMED WITH
THE WAY I AM FEELING
SO DESPERATE DEEP INSIDE
FROM MY HURT I'M DEALING

> WITH THIS AGONY AND PAIN
> THAT SITS WITH ME ALL THE TIME
> YOU MIGHT WELL THINK IT'S A GAME
> BUT DO YOU SEE ME LAUGHING?

SO OVERWHELMED WITH
THE PARANOIA INSIDE MY HEAD
SO CONSCIOUS OF THIS EVIL
FROM MY HEART THAT'S SO DEAD

> WITH THIS AGONY AND PAIN
> THAT SITS WITH ME ALL THE TIME
> YOU MIGHT WELL THINK IT'S A GAME
> BUT DO YOU SEE ME LAUGHING?

SO DISEMPOWERED BY YOUR
CONTROL OF MY EMOTIONS
SO FRIGHTENED OF THIS WAY
YOU TREAT ME INTO ISOLATION

> WITH THIS AGONY AND PAIN
> THAT SITS WITH ME ALL THE TIME
> YOU MIGHT WELL THINK IT'S A GAME
> BUT DO YOU SEE ME LAUGHING?

SO LABELLED BY YOUR

Helen Care

PIGEONHOLED DIAGNOSIS
SO UNDERMINED BY THIS
NOTION OF PROGNOSIS

WITH THIS AGONY AND PAIN
THAT SITS WITH ME ALL THE TIME
YOU MIGHT WELL THINK IT'S A GAME
BUT DO YOU SEE ME LAUGHING?

<u>MARCH 2004</u>

WITH ANGER COMES HOPE

Find a Solution

Explore your freedom
Only recently dreamed
About in childhood
Things not what they seemed

This time in your life
Where you try to witness
A bunch of adults
Fall in love I guess

Falling over
Join the revolution
Got lots of guts
To find a solution

Leave behind your home
Secure your life and love
Through this the hard part
Enjoy it's enough

So don't be jealous
For your green eyes will see
That those around you
Love relentlessly

Falling over
Join the revolution
Got lots of guts
To find a solution

October 2004

BLIND FAITH

I HOPE ONE DAY I WILL RECEIVE
INDIFFERENCE TO ALL OF THIS
I HOPE ONE DAY I'LL FEEL AT EASE
INSTEAD OF STANDING ON THIS ABYSS

Blind faith
To this I can relate
Is it my birthday?
Or not too much dismay

I HOPE ONE DAY I WILL BELIEVE
RESISTENCE TO ALL OF THIS
I HOPE ONE DAY I'LL CONCEIVE
NEW FAITH OF MINE, SUCH BLISS

Blind faith
To this I can create
Is it somewhere I can stay?
Or not as the case may say

BELIGERANCE, SUCH IGNORANCE
RELIEF WHEN I MOVE TO LEAVE
RESISTENCE SUCH TOLERANCE
TRY TO PLEASE, AM I NAÏVE?

Blind faith
To this is my trait
Is it something I can wait?
Or something I should delay?

WITH ANGER COMES HOPE

I HOPE ONE DAY I WILL SEIZE
CONSISTENCY TO MY WISH
I HOPE ONE DAY I WILL APPEASE
YOU INTO OWING WHAT YOU MISS

Blind faith
To this I can keep at bay
Is it something I can break?
Into pieces so far away

INSIGNIFICANCE SUCH A NUISANCE
DISEASE STEPS IN WHEN YOU FREEZE
SUBSISTANCE WITH SUCH DIFFERENCE
TRY TO HISS, AM I TOTALLY AMISS?

Blind faith
To this I can hate
Is it something I can tempt fate
Or is it when I should pray?!!!

JUNE 2003

Helen Care

Get In Touch With Yourself

We all need company
But a little distance helps
Take a sideways step
To avoid everyone else

For she needs to reflect
And for me to have my space
Not to take over me
Kept your distance of late

Get in touch with yourself
Accept all the offers of help
Get in touch with yourself
Get in touch with yourself

Open up your rubbish bag
Jump in and disappear
Inside of yourself
Far away from here

Come out quite new
After a spin wash or two
You flash the plastic
It's just so fantastic!!!

Get in touch with yourself
Accepts all the offers of help
Get in touch with yourself
Get in touch with yourself

September 2004

WITH ANGER COMES HOPE

Heart on My Sleeve

I can't fight the tears
That doesn't easily fall
Where's my moment of truth?
Healing starts, but it is small

Why do you misunderstand me?
Where's your level of understanding?
For I am dealing with my emotional pain
So why are you so demanding?

"Should I wear
My heart on my sleeve?
Should I tell you
What I believe?"

Need to create a balance
A temporary release valve
Adrenalin kicks in
As a response so loud

Emotional pain not seen
To the outside world
Feel so lost, I'm numb
With no ties, I'll swirl

"Should I wear
My heart on my sleeve?
Should I tell you
What I believe?"

Helen Care

Don't want to exist in this world
Where my own hate for myself
Is kept in for me to be in control
For when real hurt is dealt

Can all this be overcome?
Altered states of emotions
Self-destructive behaviour
Just leaves me in isolation

"Should I wear
My heart on my sleeve?
Should I tell you
What I believe?"

Being supportive is crucial
But I don't seek your approval
You shouldn't tolerate my
Distress that's such an upheaval

Keep all your peace offerings
Don't worry about my pain
Keep the door wide open
So I can come back again

"Should I wear
My heart on my sleeve?
Should I tell you
What I believe?"

September 2004

WITH ANGER COMES HOPE

WHAT DOES IT MATTER?
PONDER THE CLIMB, REACH THE MOUNTAIN
IT DOESN'T MAKE SENSE, DRINK FROM THE
FOUNTAIN
JUST WHEN YOUR PATIENCE RUNS THIN
ALONG COMES A MOMENT THAT YOU WILL
WIN

TAKE A PICTURE
WHAT DO YOU SEE?
WHERE WILL I GO?
WHERE WILL I BE?

USING MORE METAPHORS TO BUILD A
LADDER
TO REACH UP TO THE STARS, WHAT DOES IT
MATTER?

FEATS THAT'LL LAST, THAT'LL BE ACHIEVED
A DIFFUSION OF LOVE NEEDS TO BE
BELIEVED

TAKE A PICTURE
WHAT DO YOU SEE?
WHERE WILL I GO?
WHERE WILL I BE?

IT DOESN'T REALLY MATTER WHEN LOVE
COMES AROUND
PICTURE ALL THE FACES THAT SMILE
BEHIND A FROWN
A SEA OF BRIGHT FLAMES FROM BOTH LEFT
AND RIGHT

YOU ARE HOME AND DRY, YOU CAN SLEEP AT NIGHT

TAKE A PICTURE
WHAT DO YOU SEE?
WHERE WILL I GO?
WHERE WILL I BE?

USING MORE METAPHORS TO BUILD A LADDER
TO REACH UP TO THE STARS, WHAT DOES IT MATTER?
JUNE 2005

MAKE ME BITTER OR MAKE ME BETTER

CAN'T GO BACK TO THE PAST
I NEED TO REFLECT AND MOVE ON
WAS MY PAST LIFE GOING TOO FAST
I NEED TO BUILD ON WHAT I'VE BEGUN

USE IT ALL FOR THE GOOD
A VISION FOR MY FUTURE
I NEEDED TO KNOW WHERE I STOOD
I NEEDED A SENSE OF CLOSURE

YOU CAN'T ALWAYS BLAME IT ON THE WEATHER
MAKE ME BITTER OR MAKE ME BETTER
YOU CAN'T ALWAYS LOOK OVER YOUR SHOULDER
MAKE ME BITTER OR MAKE ME BETTER

WITH ANGER COMES HOPE

TRY AND KEEP YOUR EYES AHEAD
BUILD ON POTENTIAL AND ENERGY
THERE'S LIGHT AT THE END, YOU SAID
AT THE END OF THE TUNNEL OF MATURITY

MY FUTURE WILL EVOLVE IN ITS OWN TIME
I HAVE TO LEARN TO BE PATIENT
AND KIND TO MYSELF, THIS I'LL FIND
TO BE MY CHALLENGE, I'M CONFIDENT

YOU CAN'T ALWAYS BLAME IT ON THE WEATHER
MAKE ME BITTER OR MAKE ME BETTER
YOU CAN'T ALWAYS LOOK OVER YOUR SHOULDER
MAKE ME BITTER OR MAKE ME BETTER

MAY 2004

Helen Care

A Young Woman Of 27

A young woman of 27
Self-assured and robust
Both in body and in mind
Who'd know she'd combust?

She worked nine to five
Intelligent and cultivated
Fond of music and of art
Who'd thought she'd be annihilated?

She had an active life
Lived life to the full
Scarcely took a day off
Who'd thought she was emotional?

Then there came the breakdown
When she was admitted
A routine or a precaution
Expectations were limited

Disturbing dreams started
With peculiar intensity
She would sway wildly
On her feet, she was unsteady

For she could hardly feel
The ground beneath her
For she could hardly hear
The in-joke of laughter

Her hands would flail

WITH ANGER COMES HOPE

Backwards and forwards
She kept dropping her hands
In the name of the Lord

She became distressed
By all her nightmares
She couldn't be free
From all of their stares

A young woman of 27
Self-assured and robust
Both in body and mind
Who'd know she'd combust?

March 2005

The Story of Someone So Dear

Terror awakened her with alarming danger
That wasn't averted, instead so perverted
Her fever mounted, her love so hounded
His desire at night gave her such a fright

She became his drug that he couldn't give up
He totally disarmed her, her defences now a
blur
Her eyes turned black, rimmed with no slack
Just with stones of dust, she had no one to
trust

Her eyelids had a dark trait, her eyebrows
plucked into shape
That threw a shadow over her eyes that came
from a deeper disguise
Between his strong head and fingers so easily
led
Caressing the skin on her arm, does such
pleasure create harm?

His desire made a volcano on which she would
glow
Feeling the heat of his hands, it was too much,
all his demands
Beneath her delicate skin, he always knew
where to begin
Into the valleys of her flesh that always burned
her no less

WITH ANGER COMES HOPE

Her pain became a harsh cry, from childhood
until she'll die
Her trembling premonitions leave her making
decisions
That'll affect her sad life filled with pain and
such strife
Dust down all the unbearable and focus on
what's repairable

Flee from the eyes of the world as you watch
yourself unfurl
Now guided from all those now around you
she chose
To take their encouragement, for they're more
tolerant
And receptive to hear, the story of someone so
dear.

February 2006

Helen Care

Who She Should Be

Down the ladder where you stagger
Into the underground without a sound
Into the night with a fright
You turn round without a sound

No music for serenades, no presents for the
paid
Who try to impress in their address
To those who will listen, so hot his sweat
glistens
Speak to the converted who have already
asserted

Their practice of rituals, they protests are spiritual
Undermining her belief that she'll be set free
She re-opened her eyes, they're still there with lies
With no one to protect her, from all of this danger

He lies beside you, what will you do?
He's fallen asleep, a secret to keep?
Breathing so faint, your love he did taint
So angry and restless, you lie so motionless

His fever has peaked with one so weak
She feels his desire, can't set her on fire
She's left unfulfilled, later it will make her ill
Her anger won't melt, such rage she felt

At all their desire, her pain is on fire
Her journey so cheated, her breakdown
completed

WITH ANGER COMES HOPE

Every day and night, she couldn't see light
But now she can see who she should be.

February 2006

AWAKENED

SHE AWAKENED
AND SMILED GRATEFULLY
SHE HAD GIVEN
AND TAKEN CAREFULLY

SHE LAY THINKING, WOULD SHE SEE HIM
AGAIN?
SHE LAY WISHING, THAT SHE HADN'T GONE
INSANE!
SHE WAS TALKING ABOUT HER CHILDHOOD
SHE WAS MELTING LIKE SNOW, SHE WOULD

FILL THE IDYLLIC SCENE, THEN REFUSE TO
LEAVE
AN ATMOSPHERE SO PURE, SHE IS NEVER
QUITE SURE
IF SHE EVER WANT'S TO BE WITH SOMEONE
SO FREE
FROM ALL OF HER PAIN, YOU'LL FIND SHE'LL
GAIN

PEACE WITHIN HER HEART THAT WON'T
EVER DEPART
OR ABANDON HER SOUL, INSTEAD SHE'LL
FEEL WHOLE
SHE WON'T BE OFFENDED IF YOU
PRETENDED
TO CARE FOR HER, YOUR LOVE SO
DEFERRED

WITH ANGER COMES HOPE

IT WAS YOU'RE WORDS THAT WERE SO
ABSURD
SHE FEELS SO CONFUSED AND WITH
EVERYTHING TO LOSE
IS IT TIME TO CONFESS, FACE UP TO THIS
MESS
WITH ALL OF YOUR DEMANDS, SHE'LL WRING
YOUR HANDS

UNTIL THEY FALL OFF, FOR SHE'S HAD
ENOUGH
THE BLOOD IN YOUR VEINS MAKE HER FEEL
FAINT
SHE WAS SO TALKATIVE WONDERING IF
SHE'D FORGIVE
WILL HER SENSITIVITY MELT YOU WITH HOW
SHE FELT

SHE AWAKENED
AND SMILED GRATEFULLY
SHE HAD GIVEN
AND TAKEN CAREFULLY

FEBRUARY 2006

Helen Care

On The Surface

Attraction only becomes
A deep-rooted desire
When you breathe someone
In and ignite their fire

Find their essence appealing
Interaction tends to happen
On a subconscious level
So keep your face deadpan

Many of us remain unaware
For we struggle with relationships
That appears perfect on paper
But never really on the inner layer

No one tells us the facts of life
Are partners really compatible?
Please go easy on the perfume
For we are all acutely vulnerable

Personal chemistry is individual
It gets more refined as we age
May be we need more guidance
Ideally read on and turn the page

Many of us remain unaware
For we struggle with relationships
That appears perfect on paper
But never really on the inner layer

February 2005

WITH ANGER COMES HOPE

LOVE OR LUST

She didn't immediately realise her enthusiasm
was so wild
She wanted a good bit of romance; a few sessions
left her in a trance
Forward looking and generous, he even helped
but was nervous
Giving birth is such a bombshell, is a disability a
living hell?

She became unable to focus on anything else she
would choke
Feed her endless cups of tea and listen to her
every anxiety
Life did not improve it simply changed
Total dependency, never rearranged

For at the centre of her life was this child so full of
light
Agonised at parting with her, for she was her only
daughter
She ploughed back into routine to escape from
where she had been
Along came more children, a sense of guilt was
building

Living in each other's shoes, pushed limits,
missed the clues
Feeling desolate when he left, remembering back
to when they met
She was ashamed at feeling so emotional with
such meaning

Helen Care

Her pain just became worse, even more than
giving birth

Now he has moved in with you, such betrayal
leaves her blue
So many scenes she's blocked out, her memories
just leave her with doubt
All those years, of your trust
Now betrayed by love or lust?

March 2006

WITH ANGER COMES HOPE

Please Just Hold Her

**You look like you have
The weight of the world
On your shoulders
Please just hold her**

And for who can blame her?
With this impending carnage
With a meltdown on the horizon
Dig deep and look for a bridge

To provide an escape route
To question your soul searching
Within time you will leave
Looking so troubled, you're hurting

Clutching onto the straws of life
It's hard to tell or understand
Is life a celebration or test?
You're so desperate to demand

You know that it's no surprise
Being miserable is so unkind
Endure a slew of comparisons
To ghosts from back in time

For there's far more going on
Than appears on the surface
Flirt with life and fly the flag
Promoting experience in a crisis

A life so kind but directionless

Helen Care

Rambling on what could persuade
The push and shove that hurts
When it cuts with a razor blade

**You look like you have
The weight of the world
On your shoulders
Please just hold her**

<u>February 2005</u>

WITH ANGER COMES HOPE

<u>Witness</u>

**"I was a witness to all of this
What can I cling on to?
Memories twist in my stomach
Who can I turn to?"**

You've always had a lot of nerve
For you always tried to choose
To bring out your hurt and pain
For what do you have to lose?

Will we ever find some common ground?
Somewhere to find some peace
That will bring some freedom
To express myself and end the lease

You've always had a lot of nerve
All you bought, all you paid for
We never had any common ground
Never respected me, just slaughtered

Holding onto the pain
That lies beneath
Try not to refrain
Give it your release

Living within your fear
Is not living at all
So start to climb
Before you fall

"I was a witness to all of this

What can I cling on to?
Memories twist in my stomach
Who can I turn to?"

January 2005

WITH ANGER COMES HOPE

Getting Better

Getting better, getting better
You were torn apart, with a broken heart

By someone you trusted, by someone you loved
Thought they cared, this is all too much
Some day's you'd cry, some day's you hoped
For a true way out, to be able to cope

Please help the knots in her tummy go away
Help her settle down and help her feel okay
Muddled up feelings, she'd paint and write
To express her emotions she's had all her life

In years to come she really does hope
To love life again and laugh at the joke
She's looking forward to the rest of her life
With encouragement, she'll overcome this strife

Through the doors that are now open
She can start again, she won't be broken

Getting better, getting better
You were torn apart, with a broken heart

July 2006

79

Helen Care

So Much Fun!!!!!!!!!

You wake up one morning
Confident about your ability
To solve all the problems
In your life so rewardingly

Achieve all your ambitions
Proving not to being temporary
Your feelings turn into obsessions
As each day passes relentlessly

Your mind is clearer
Your instincts sharper
You see solutions reliably
With a frightening clarity

You act on this feeling
A performance in every way
Become more charismatic
And confident, so dramatic

So completely in control
Of events and relationships
That shapes your life
Brush aside every blip

Those who urge caution
Are just whingers who
Do not know how to play
Life's game right on cue

Your spending increases

WITH ANGER COMES HOPE

As you, follow your instinct
Accumulate to speculate
But bring you to the brink

Things you wanted to buy
Experiences you wanted to indulge
Are there for you to acquire
Free from constraints that'll solve

Petty daily nuisances
That has held you back
Is there something wrong?
Is there something that you lack?

Feelings of dis-inhibition
At simply where you begun
They are just too enjoyable
You've never had so much fun!!!!

September 2006

81

Helen Care

Between Here and There

People are not ready to accept
That you can rise up from the ashes
From being committed for your own good
When they're frightened of their own crisis

Sat in my seminar of education
When a tidal wave washed me away
Totally obliterating my little world
For a few minutes of sanity, I went crazy

Looking down on this scary situation
To see if anyone is listening to me
But they are all engrossed in their
Own point of view with no such empathy

I rush out and end up in the nearest pub
I've lost count of how many drinks I had
Got on the phone searching for help
This situation sickens me and makes me sad

Most people here pass over my validation
To be an equal who deserves respect
Performing perforations of my creditability
Their sense of me being a threat is something I
detect

Between here and there
Until an opening exists
Threatening those in power
An opening they can't resist

WITH ANGER COMES HOPE

LOVEABLE

BRING ME BACK TO THE NEXT DAY
THEN CONFESS I HEAR YOU SAY
WALK TOWARDS THE SEA AND SAND
LAY YOUR CLAIMS TO ALL THIS LAND

YOU RESPOND FROM THE CORE
SO SENSUAL AND SO PURE
YOU'RE AMAZED AND ALWAYS KIND
YOUR FREEDOM YOU CANNOT HIDE

SO LIBERATE WHAT'S TOO MUCH
YOU'RE ANXIETIES YOU CANNOT TOUCH
SHE'S SO IMPULSIVE BUT IRRESISTABLE
SHE'S SO COMPULSIVE BUT LOVEABLE

TIME AT SEA, THE SUN AND MOON
BRIGHTEN HER LIFE, NEVER CAME TOO
SOON
NOW IN THE CITY OF ORANGE AUTUMN
LOVE WILL VANISH BEHIND THE SUN

BEFORE YOU ARRIVE, FIND YOUR KEY
TO OPEN THE DOOR TO SET YOU FREE
SO FULL OF RESERVE AND SYMPATHY
FOR WHAT I LOST SO WRECKLESSLY

VOICE YOUR RESPECT OF WHAT'S INSPIRED
YOU TO COMPOSE, EMOTIONS YOU FIRED
SHE'S SO IMPULSIVE BUT IRRESISTABLE
SHE'S SO COMPULSIVE BUT LOVEABLE
FEBRUARY 2006

So Relaxed and Now Happy

**She opened her eyes, brought on by a surprise
She's liberated and free, so relaxed and now
happy**

Free from so much to enjoy his love
With a warm heart we're never far apart
She glazed at her stranger lying naked beside her
Like a statute of shame, she didn't want to touch
again

He resembled her anger, regretting all the danger
Detached and disentangled, a moment frozen and
strangled
Hesitation, exhalation
Slide softly out of bed, escape while he slept

She closed her eyes, so blind to all his lies
She's tired and caught, so anxious and now
fraught
On the shelf there's powder and lipstick in the
shower
She smiled at them and she thought again

Contemplate these objects without the slightest
regrets
With envy or jealously based on her dependency...
on...
Her capacity for pain, she breathed in again
She felt deep pleasure in stealing his treasure

While combing her hair she would sit and stare

WITH ANGER COMES HOPE

While enjoying his home, this is a danger zone
Her eyes now blind to everything silent
She once loved but never touched

She opened her eyes, brought on by a surprise
She's liberated and free, so relaxed and now
happy

February 2006

Helen Care

Tumbling

It began with a headache
And lasted for a lifetime
Struck down by pressure
Of sexuality, so sublime

I was suffering
I was falling
In and out of
Tumbling

I was in shock
Incomprehensible
I was so upset
So vulnerable

It was like being under water
I can't hear anything at all
Not in control of my movements
I can't understand the world

It felt as though I was trapped
It felt dark under the surface
I didn't know how to get out
I didn't know how to find the trace

I was suffering
I was falling
In and out of
Tumbling

I was in shock

WITH ANGER COMES HOPE

Incomprehensible
I was so upset
So vulnerable

January 2005

Helen Care

Just Swallow Me Whole

Just swallow me whole
As I am out of control
Hug me, as I feel cold
Please will you steal my soul?

I don't like my existence
So why are you so persistent?
For me to try and change
My life that feels so strange

I need protection
Not rejection
Hold me close
When I feel low

Please will you steal my soul?
Hug me, as I feel cold
As I am out of control
Just swallow me whole

April 2006

WITH ANGER COMES HOPE

LEARN HOW TO FEEL

I FEEL PAIN HOWLING IN EVERY PART OF ME
I FEEL SO CHEATED I'M LEFT FEELING
ANGRY
OUT OF THE SHADOWS NEXT TIME WHEN WE
MEET
SHOUTING AT YOUR VOICES AS YOU
SHUFFLE YOUR FEET

SO ANXIOUS AND AFRAID, ARE YOU ABLE
TO GIVE
THE RECOGNITION I CRAVE TO ENABLE ME
TO LIVE
NO FAULT OF YOUR OWN YOU HAD TO
ENDURE
FEELING SO ALONE AND NOT TOO SURE

ACCIDENTS CAN HAPPEN TO THE MIND AND
BODY
AND THE CONSEQUENCES LEAVE ME
FEELING SORRY
THERE IS NO DOUBT TO THIS DARK CAUSE
SO SOCIALLY ATTRACTIVE YIELDING SUCH
APPLAUSE

IF ONLY THERE WAS A CURE TO OUR INNER
ANGUISH
SUCH SATISFACTION LEAVES ME
SQUEEMISH
SUCH HAUNTING IMAGERY, SUCH HUMOUR
AND SKILL

Helen Care

**SUSPENSE AND EXCITEMENT, BEAUTY IS
SUCH A THRILL**

**SUCH AN ODDESSY OF HOPE, FIND MY LOST
MIND
WHERE I HOLD MY LOVE, NEVER BITTER
ALWAYS KIND
LIFE IS A CHALLENGE, THE CLUES ARE
REAL
COMFORT MY MIND AND LEARN HOW TO
FEEL**

MAY 2006

WITH ANGER COMES HOPE

<u>DARKNESS IN HER HEAD</u>

SUSPEND THE LAW OF PHYSICS
FOR WHAT GOES UP DOES NOT
NECESSARILY COME DOWN
DARKNESS IN HER HEAD IS HER LOT

ALWAYS ATTEMPTING TO GET SOME REST
A STATE OF MIND SHE MAY NEVER FIND
PLAGUED BY MONSTERS AND NIGHTMARES
FOR HER REALITY IS NEVER KIND

**FOR TIME MAY RUN ROUND IN CIRCLES
FLOATING IN THE DARKNESS IN HER HEAD
SKIPPING BETWEEN NOW AND THEN
FLOATING IN THE DARKNESS IN HER HEAD**

TICKING CLOCKS, BLANK FACES WITH
FLOWERS
THESE ARE ALL THINGS YOU CAN GO BACK
TO
INVISIBLE TO THOSE VOICES THAT
SURROUND
SEE THE WORLD WITH EYES BRAND NEW

HER WORLD LOOKS HUGE AND MENACING
QUIVERING LIKE A MOUNTAIN OF JELLY
LIKE A PLANET SPINNING IN ITS ORBIT
EITHER WAY A DISCOUNTED YELLING

**FOR TIME MAY RUN ROUND IN CIRCLES
FLOATING IN THE DARKNESS IN HER HEAD
SKIPPING BETWEEN NOW AND THEN**

Helen Care

FLOATING IN THE DARKNESS IN HER HEAD

<u>FEBRUARY 2004</u>

WITH ANGER COMES HOPE

KEEPS ME ALIVE

GETTING IN TOUCH WITH
FEELING THE EMOTIONS
FOR THIS PAIN INSIDE
KEEPS ME ALIVE

SO OVERWHELMED
I DON'T NEED TO TELL
YOU ARE MY HELL
INTO MY PAST YOU DELVE

RESIST THE TEMPTATION
TO SEEK YOUR LOVE
THIS IS FAR TOO MUCH
REJECTION IN ISOLATION

SO DISAPPOINTED IN ME
BY MY BEHAVIOUR
NOT BELIEVING IN YOUR SAVIOUR
DAMNED TO HELL FOR ETERNITY

WHAT HAPPENED TO LOVE?
NOT IN ENDLESS SUPPLY
FULL OF HURT AND LIES
I HAVE BEEN FAILED BY GOD

A REQUEST FOR APOLOGIES
FOR MY LACK OF RESPECT
ANIMOSITY IS WHAT I SUSPECT
BLUDGENING MY VULNERABILITIES

Helen Care

GETTING IN TOUCH WITH
FEELING THE EMOTIONS
FOR THIS PAIN INSIDE
KEEPS ME ALIVE

<u>MAY 2004</u>

WITH ANGER COMES HOPE

A Sense of Movement

A chemical change
A fizz bomb on my tongue
Explodes the battle in me
Putting to rest feeling wrong

A gateway to sleep
Bombed out to get rest
No waking nightmares
I wake up feeling my best

**A sense of movement
A sense of progress
Feeling myself again
Reflect upon my distress**

I want to move on
I want to become
Someone, someone
That I want to become

Completely unique
Complete with mystique
That makes me neat
Want to feel complete

**A sense of movement
A sense of progress
Feeling myself again
Reflect upon my distress**

October 2004

Helen Care

MY GUIDING STAR

HI THERE YOU FIRESTARTER

WHAT WOULD I DO WITHOUT YA?

WOULD WE STILL SET UP HOME?

WOULD WE? ONLY HEAVEN KNOWS

FOR YOU ARE MY GUIDING STAR

DOESN'T MATTER WHERE YOU ARE

I FEEL SAFE WHEN YOU'RE AROUND

WHEN I THINK OF YOU I FEEL PROUD

FROM FEELING FULL OF FEAR

TO WELLING UP WITH TEARS

THINKING OF YOU ALWAYS HELPS

WHEN I AM JUST BY MYSELF

WHAT I'M TRYING TO SAY

IS I MISS YOU EVERYDAY

WITH ANGER COMES HOPE

ALL THOSE HUGS AND KISSES

ALL THOSE LOVE WISHES

YOU ARE ALWAYS IN MY THOUGHTS

YOU ARE ALWAYS IN MY DREAMS

YOU ARE ALWAYS IN MY HEART

I LOVE YOU ALWAYS, DON'T EVER LET US
PART

DECEMBER 2002

FRIENDS AND MUSIC

As I put another record on, I think about a time
When I felt so alone, lost in music I'd find
A place I could be, most content and
Safe in the sound of music's hand
That rocked my cradle with such innocence
That reached my core giving me deliverance

Friends and music
Are such a comfort
I'm feeling safe
From all hurt

The energy of sound inspired my creativity
Putting a voice to my songs of reality
Chapters of my life hold no glory
As I unravel my troubled story
As I now reflect, others can see
My troubled life in their own journey

Friends and music
Are such a comfort
I'm feeling safe
From all hurt

October 2004

WITH ANGER COMES HOPE

Anybody's Lover

You phone to say you're coming round
And then take all day to arrive
You say you've brought a video to watch
But you've seen it already, you lied

**Watch, then look and chill out
We don't need to fight anymore
Sex, sleep and pleasant dreams
We don't need to keep a score**

You say that you'll stay the night
But then you walk out the door
You wish me a night of sweet dreams
But the nightmares haunt me once more

You said that you loved me
But I don't believe you anymore
What you say and what you do
Don't match up to being adored

**Watch, then look and chill out
We don't need to fight anymore
Sex, sleep and pleasant dreams
We don't need to keep a score**

You say one thing to me
When you actually mean another
I really don't want this game
For I can't be anybody's lover

March 2005

CHOOSE TO REFUSE

PLEASE WILL YOU REFRAIN
FROM MAKING YOUR ADVANCES
IT'S LIKE GIVING UP CIGARETTES
CRAVINGS STIFLE MY CHANCES

WHAT GIVES YOU THE RIGHT
TO IMPOSE YOUR FANTASIES
UPON YOUR FIRST BORN CHILD
TOO YOUNG FOR SUCH TRAVESTIES

"Strangled her right to say no
Thwarted as you steeped so low
No respect for her is no excuse
She has the right to choose to refuse"

YES, TOO YOUNG FOR SEX GAMES
ALWAYS ATTENTIVE TO YOUR DEMANDS
STUCK IN A VICIOUS CYCLE OF
VIOLATIONS THAT SHOULD BE BANNED

CLOSE ON BECOMING A PAEDOPHILE
EXPLOITED FOR SEXUAL GRATIFICATION
FOR SHE WAS ONLY A YOUNG CHILD
YOU SHOULD BE SUBJECT TO CASTRATION

"Strangled her right to say no
Thwarted as you steeped so low
No respect for her is no excuse
She has the right to choose to refuse"

FUELLED BY MISGUIDED LOVE

WITH ANGER COMES HOPE

INCEST ON SUCH A GRAND SCALE
NOT ABLE TO SAY ENOUGH IS ENOUGH
IN YOUR LOVE FOR HER, YOU DID FAIL...

... HER, WITH HER RIGHT TO CHOOSE TO
REFUSE
YES, HER RIGHT TO CHOOSE TO REFUSE...

SEPTEMBER 2003

Violent and Unkind (Part 2)

Have you ever faced death?
When it's staring back at your face
Threatened within an inch of your life
Might as well slit my throat with a knife

Have you ever faced death?
When surrounded by violence
Outnumbered by three to one
Threatening me without a conscience

I've never been so scared
Since I was a young child
Fear with traumatic dread
Pain so violent and unkind

It's not just the violence you know
For such invasion screws you up
Dirty, violated and so defiled
Such an experience of grave hurt

They say that it's such a violent act
Power over women into humiliation
Like having sex with an audience
I think not, just left in isolation

Have you ever faced death?
When surrounded by violence
Outnumbered by three to one
Threatening me without a conscience

I've never been so scared

WITH ANGER COMES HOPE

Since I was a young child
Fear with traumatic dread
Pain so violent and unkind

__April 2004__

Helen Care

IN A BLANKET WITH MY HEART

LOOK AROUND AND SEE

THE COLOURS IN THE ROOM

THE SHAPE OF THINGS TO COME

PEOPLE NEARBY YOU ASSUME

LISTEN TO THE SOUNDS

AROUND YOU, YOUR BREATHING

TRAFFIC, BIRDS AND PEOPLE

FEEL YOUR BODY LEAVING...

...YOU BEHIND...BE UNKIND

ALWAYS TRYING, NOW I'M FLYING

TOUCH YOUR ARMS AND LEGS

SIT ON THE CHAIR OR FLOOR

THAT SUPPORTS YOUR DISTRESS

YOUR BREATHING YOU CAN'T IGNORE

WITH ANGER COMES HOPE

TELL YOURSELF YOU'RE OKAY

FEEL THE FEELINGS

YOU'RE SAFE AND NOW OUT OF DANGER

DON'T DENY YOUR HEALING... THAT
LEAVES...

...

...YOU BEHIND... BE UNKIND

ALWAYS TRYING, NOW I'M FLYING

WHERE DID I LEAVE?

AND NOW WHERE DO I START?

WRAP MY EMOTIONS TIGHTLY

IN A BLANKET WITH MY HEART

<u>SEPTEMBER 2004</u>

It's So Comforting

> **It's so comforting**
> **To know you are there**
> **For me when I'm down**
> **And full up with despair**

My insecurities don't measure up
To your endless patience of me
When I'm angry and so confused
And not really feeling in reality

My frustrations don't faze you
As you, lift me up so lovingly
As I always, try to push boundaries
You support the fence with consistency

> **It's so comforting**
> **To know you are there**
> **For me when I'm down**
> **And full up with despair**

My tolerance of pain tells you
What I need to survive and grow
Your encouragement and support
For me to build on your faith you know

My endless need of reassurance
Grounds me into feeling safe
When you tell me, you're here for me
Finding my soul hasn't come too late

> **It's so comforting**

WITH ANGER COMES HOPE

To know you are there
For me when I'm down
And full up with despair

September 2004

Helen Care

`I WISH…

I WISH I'D LEFT MY FINGERPRINTS SOMEWHERE

SO THAT I COULDN'T BE FOUND

GUILTY OF CARRYING GUILTY SECRETS

CHANGE MY NUMBER AND FEEL THE GROUND

I WISH I'D LEFT MY ENEMIES SOMEWHERE

SO THAT I COULDN'T BE TORMENTED

IN CHAINS SO BRUTAL AND TERRIFYING

CHANGE MY THOUGHTS AND NOT FEEL DEMENTED

I want to stand up on my own

All those devils are unbeknown

For I will have the strength

To rise above with such depth

I WISH I'D LEFT MY HEART SOMEWHERE

WITH ANGER COMES HOPE

SO THAT I COULDN'T FALL IN LOVE

WITH FEELINGS SO STRONG AND
CONFUSING

CHANGE MY EMOTIONS IS NOT ENOUGH

I WISH I'D LEFT MY HURT SOMEWHERE

SO THAT I COULDN'T GET UPSET

SO EASILY OVERWHELMED AND INSECURE

CHANGE MY LIFE OR IS IT OVER YET?

Trying to find love and peace

Yearning for your release

Feed me to the lions and tigers

You should know I'm a fighter

JUNE 2003

Reaching For Love

The healing is
Coming to terms
With emotions that
Are lessons to learn

A second skin
That I wear beneath
Makes me feel safe
So deep and at ease

**The will to
Rise above
For I won't tire
On reaching for love**

Taking time out
To take good stock
Such concentration
On how to unlock

Now I see the light
Bubbling like champagne
Living is this journey
While I consolidate

**The will to
Rise above
For I won't tire
On reaching for love**

WITH ANGER COMES HOPE

Friends are precious
Others too are friends
Too precious to let go
Like learning life's lessons

October 2004

In Our Relationship

Social butterflies
Kind but lonely
Beautiful wings
And very friendly

I'm over you
So I won't stay
Then you'll notice
Get your own way

An anxiety attack
Undermines happiness
I felt left out
With this distress

Ridiculously brilliant
A best friendship
A better headspace
In our relationship

Will it be cool?
Will it work out?
It's been wonderful
You know I can't doubt

I broke down
I cried and cried
In the back seat
To avoid the ride

Broke her heart

WITH ANGER COMES HOPE

Couldn't be there
Help me up to a
Better anywhere

**Ridiculously brilliant
A best friendship
A better headspace
In our relationship**

November 2004

Helen Care

<u>MY FLOWER</u>

I DON'T THINK I'M DISTURBED
AS YOU THINK I SHOULD BE
FOR I AM WELL AWARE
OF MY DREADFUL REALITY

**IT'S AS THOUGH IT WASN'T ME
A FILM WITH A NEW ACTRESS
DEPICTING SCENE BY SCENE
THE REALITY I CAN'T ASSESS**

HOW DID THIS ALL HAPPEN?
WHERE WAS MY SENSE OF CALM?
THEIR WHITE LIGHT BURNS MY SOUL
UNTIL NOW I RAISE THE ALARM

**WHY DID THE SYSTEM
REPLACE MY PROMISCUITY?
THAT FOLLOWED ON FROM
MY ABUSIVE HISTORY**

I THINK I ONCE WAS, A
FLOWER OF INNER BEAUTY
BUT MY BLACK HEART
TAINTED MY VULNERABILITY

**SO FULL OF BOBBING PETALS
THAT REST ON MY FLOWER
FROM SEEDS SO DAMAGED
MY FIGHT BACK I EMPOWER**

<u>MAY 2004</u>

LEAVE THIS BEHIND

SHE WAS A NORMAL CHILD

SAME AS ANY OTHER CHILD

HAPPY.... HAPPY

FROM OUTGOING TO A HEAP

FRIGHTENED OF THE DARK

SCARED TO GO TO SLEEP

HE WAS A FRIENDLY FACE

A MASTER OF DISGUISE

HE TIED A RIBBON AROUND HER

A TRUST SHE WAS DENIED

SHE HOPED THAT THE SECRET

WOULD COME OUT AT LAST

DOWNHILL... DOWNHILL

COMFORT EATING, FEELING LOW

SHE JUST COULDN'T SLEEP

SCARED TO CRY YOU KNOW

Helen Care

HE WAS A FRIENDLY FACE

A MASTER OF DISGUISE

HE TIED A RIBBON AROUND HER

A TRUST SHE WAS DENIED

SHE JUST COULDN'T COPE

SO SHE TRIED TO TELL

SCARY... SCARY

SHE'LL LEAVE THIS BEHIND

FACING FEARS ALL THE TIME

SHE'LL LEAVE THIS BEHIND

JUNE 2002

WITH ANGER COMES HOPE

JESUS ON T.V.

Feeling so emotional
Feeling so distressed
Demand to know my name
Denial of my request

Hostile and unhelpful
Every time I tried to say
Talk all over me again and
Again... no empathy

Screaming from the inside
Why aren't you listening to me?
Need to seek refuge again
Jesus on TV. Jesus on TV.

Why are you so quick to judge?
I feel angry most of the time
If you understood at all
Then you'd realise

Pick myself up again
Feeling lower than before
I really need some help now
You should know the score

Screaming from the inside
Why aren't you listening to me?
Need to seek refuge again
Jesus on TV. Jesus on TV.

Emotionally distressed at your request

Helen Care

Unhelpful to say, no empathy again
Judging me all the time, so understand to realise
Up again like before helps lower the score

Screaming from the inside
Why aren't you listening to me?
Need to seek refuge again
Jesus on TV. Jesus on TV.

April 2002 / 2006

WITH ANGER COMES HOPE

LIKE LIFE

LIFE IS SO FRAGILE
    ICY COLD

LIKE DROWNING SKIES
    BURNING HOT

LIKE WEEPING TREES
    FALLING STARS

I'M GLAD TO BE ALIVE
    READY OR NOT

LIFE IS SO FRAGILE
    BLACK SOOT

YOU'RE ON TENDER HOOKS
    DRY SAND

LIKE FALLING STARS
    FLAKES OF SNOW

I'M GLAD OF YOUR LOOKS
    READY TO LAND

LIFE IS SO FRAGILE
    WET RAIN

LIKE AN ECLIPSED MOON
    GREY CLOUDS

LIKE BURNING SAND
    CUTTING WIND

I'M GLAD TO SEE YOU SOON
    READY OR PROUD

LIFE IS SO FRAGILE
    SHINING MOON

LIKE A DULL MORNING
    FEEL THE DRAFT

LIKE A SPINNING SUN
    WINDS OF CHANGE

I'M GLAD OF THE WARMING
    READY TO LAUGH

LIFE IS SO FRAGILE
    THUNDER CLAPS

LIKE A LISTENING NIGHT
    HEAVY RAIN

LIKE CRYSTAL RAIN
    SOAKING WET

I'M GLAD YOU SEE THE LIGHT
    READY AGAIN

WITH ANGER COMES HOPE

LIFE IS SO FRAGILE
        SUNNY DAY

LIKE A FADING LIGHT
        COLD NIGHT

LIKE ONE LAST BREATH
        REALITY CHECKS

I'M GLAD YOU LIKE LIFE
        LIKE LIFE

OCTOBER 2002

PROTECTION

ARTICULATE AND DETERMINED
IN DEFENCE OF HER PRINCIPLES
DESPITE ATTEMPTS TO BEAT HER
INTO SUBMISSION SHE STILL INSTILLS

HER MIND IS VERY PRECISE
ALWAYS GIVING AN EXACT REPLY
SHE IS NOT LIKE ALL THE OTHERS
SHE REALLY HASN'T LOST HER MIND

A REPLY THAT WARRANTS AN ANSWER
WITH RESPECT AND BLATANT COURTESY
HER SILENCE HAS BEEN INCREASED
A LACK OF FREEDOM-LIVE OR LET IT BE

JUSTICE NOT REVENGE
NEED TOUGHER CONTROLS
STAMP OUT THIS TORTURE
NO EXCUSE FOR THEIR ROLES

NOT A CRISIS RESPONSE
TO HUMAN VIOLATIONS
RESPONDING TO THEIR HURTS
CHILDREN NEED PROTECTION

FROM PEOPLE LIKE YOU
YOU KNOW WHO YOU ARE
JUSTICE WILL CATCH UP WITH YOU
YOU WON'T ESCAPE VERY FAR!!!

SEPTEMBER 2003

RUN OUT OF TIME

WHAT THE HELL
DOES HE WANT?
FOR MY MEMORIES
SOLIDIFY INTO ONE LUMP

I'M PRETTY CONFUSED
I'M UNDER PRESSURE
I CAN'T FOCUS ON
MY NEW ADVENTURE

WHY CAN'T LIFE
BE ONE LONG PARTY?
BUT I DON'T CARE
AS I'M NOW OVER THIRTY

YOU WERE THE QUIET TYPE
IN A CROWD SO SMALL
WISHING TO BE ON MY OWN
PLAYING GAMES I RECALL

ONE DAY, IN DESPERATION
I TOOK A ROLL OF TAPE
AND PATCHED UP MY WOUNDS
SO EXPLICIT OF MY HATE

A RED LINE NOW DIVIDES US
SPLITS THE ROOM INTO TWO
FROM NOW ON DON'T DARE
TO CROSS OVER LIKE YOU DO

FOR THIS IS MY SIDE

Helen Care

DON'T CROSS THE LINE
PLEASE DON'T BOTHER ME
AS I'VE RUN OUT OF TIME

<u>MAY 2004</u>

WITH ANGER COMES HOPE

Up To My Neck

You look like
You're having a seizure
You lurch forward
Stop trying to please her

Your head's shaking
Your eyes scrunched
Your tight lips
Refuse to eat lunch

Your mouth punctuates
Your word's jabbing
Your finger at me
Now who's laughing?

I need another point of view
To give me a reality check
I don't want to be marooned
In the sand and up to my neck

For you're not having
An epileptic fit
For your dancing
Without being rhythmic

You've a feel for youth
With their electronics
Only to be demolished
With motions so spasmodic

You've such epic scope

Helen Care

Harking back to the days
When your self confidence
Drifted off into a haze

I need another point of view
To give me a reality check
I don't want to be marooned
In the sand and up to my neck

October 2004

WITH ANGER COMES HOPE

RESCUE ME

I NEED SOMETHING TO EAT

SHE'S YELLING AT THEM TOO

STOMPING DOWN THE HALLWAY

NOT KNOWING WHAT SHE'LL DO

I DIP MY HANDS BACK IN THE WATER

SCALDING, BURNING, IT'S TOO LATE

SHE CATCHES ME OUT AGAIN

AN ALMIGHTY BLOW TO MY FACE

RESCUE ME, RESCUE ME

OH, WHY CAN'T I BE RESCUED?

RESCUE ME, RESCUE ME

ISN'T MY TIME OF RESCUE OVERDUE?

I TOPPLE DOWN ON TO THE FLOOR

NOT A SINGLE LOOK OF DEFIANCE

Helen Care

AVOID HER LOOKS AND SCREAMS

ANOTHER BLOW FOR MY SILENCE

CHOKING ON MY TEARS OF DEFEAT

SHE SEEMED SATISFIED AT LAST

COUNT HER STEPS OF RETREAT

A SICH OF RELIEF FROM THE PAST

RESCUE ME, RESCUE ME

OH, WHY CAN'T I BE RESCUED?

RESCUE ME, RESCUE ME

ISN'T MY TIME OF RESCUE OVERDUE?

JANUARY 2003

WITH ANGER COMES HOPE

MIDDLE GROUND

ALL THAT GUILT ALL THAT BLAME

ALL THAT HURT, FEELING FULL OF SHAME

        Violence and hate

        Help came too late

        The legacy lives on

        Anger's already begun

ALL THAT FEAR, ALL THAT SEX

ALL THAT LOVE, FEARFUL OF WHAT NEXT

ALL THOSE STORIES, ALL THOSE LIES

ALL THOSE WORDS, FEELINGS I CAN'T HIDE

ALL THAT JAZZ, ALL THAT COVER-UP

ALL THAT DECEIT, FEELING SO INCOMPLETE

Helen Care

Trying to find a middle ground

Let go of feelings that abound

Trying to find a middle ground

My heart was lost, never found

FEBRUARY 2003

WITH ANGER COMES HOPE

<u>Inner</u>

Inner churning
In turmoil
Inside out
My blood boils

Inner writhing
Much anxiety
So confused
My insecurity

Inner pain
Really hurts
My blame
Be alert

Inner loss
On my own
Desperation
Feel alone

Inner peace
Let him go
A new future
A new flow

Inner soul
Find myself
New domain
So heartfelt

Inner heart

That beats
New pulse
Won't deceive?

March 2005

WITH ANGER COMES HOPE

Runaway

Vulnerable children
Running away from home
Not even reported missing
No wonder they feel alone

Some are sleeping rough
Putting themselves at risk
Of violence and sexual
Assault and then dismissed

To a life of misery
To a life of insecurity
Please don't pass them by
Reach out to understand why

That could be your child
Except they've lost their smile
Struggling from one day
To the next, unperplexed

Who knows? Who cares?
Where they exist
Not even reported
Not even missed

Sleeping rough at night
A risky lifestyle
To support themselves
Each one only a child

We need to listen and see, for

Helen Care

While they keep the demons at bay
In a sea of pain and uncertainty
Do you ever see the runaway?

So open up your eyes
Observe these childhood lives
Hurt has led them astray
A statistic, another runaway

May 2007

WITH ANGER COMES HOPE

The Urge to Be Real

Drowning in an ocean
In a torrent of hurt
Trying to stay afloat
I have to stay alert

Drowning in the ebb and flow
That rushes to my head
High on emotion and love
Much more than I said

Bobbing up and down
On a wave that rushes
Me up and then under
Floating as my mouth gushes

To scream out for help
To shout to be heard
To sink with the pain
That I try to defer

Far away from me
I don't want to feel
As I will fall under
The urge to be real

March 2005

Helen Care

She was devilishly beautiful
Always immaculately dressed
Such a perfectionist in her life
What did she expect?

She could be very loving
At the same, time very strict
Manipulative and egocentric
A depressive needing a fix

She did everything at 90mph
Or not at all, sitting still
Her arrogance stopped her
From tackling problems at will

She could be a lot of fun
But I was frightened by her
She taught me much, but
Damaged me on way with her laughter

She wanted control of everything
How I looked and how I dressed
Who my friends and partners were
Having to be your way that was best

This criticism has stayed with me
For I am now my own worst enemy
Massively insecure of myself, but
It wasn't just me, but also everyone else!!!

October 2004

136

WITH ANGER COMES HOPE

Release

The thoughts flood
I sit and freeze
Memories overwhelm
Like a bad dream

Back in that place
So evil and unkind
Relive the nightmare
That serves to undermine

Start to disconnect
Can't stand the pain
That's too hurtful
And full of shame

Unspeakable acts
Serve to denigrate
An innocent child
Who tried to pray

To find an escape
From all this Hell
Of sex and desire
Need someone to tell

I need someone to hear
To try and rescue me
Wave a magic wand
Leave this reality

I need someone to feel

Helen Care

The pain within me
Touch me with your hand
So that I might see

I still feel haunted
Exorcise my ghosts
So that I can heal
And give me hope

Hope for my future
To feel at peace
Free from emotions
That I need to release

June 2005

WITH ANGER COMES HOPE

<u>SUCH A TONIC</u>

I ASK TOO MANY QUESTIONS

YOU SAY I DON'T LIKE THE ANSWERS

WHAT I HEAR AND WHAT I SAY

LABELS AND GUILT ARE ON THEIR WAY

BELIEVE, BELIEVE, BELIEVE, BELIEVE ME

BELIEVE ME WHEN I TELL YOU

WHEN I'VE ASKED LOTS OF PEOPLE

YOU'RE NOT EVIL OR DEMONIC

HEARING THIS - IS SUCH A TONIC

SELF-HARM AND MENTAL ILLNESS

ARE DUE TO BEING DISTRESSED

AND IN AN EMOTIONAL HOLE

ISOLATED, DOWN AND COLD

I GET STRONGER EVERY SINGLE DAY

MATURITY AND GROWTH ARE ON THEIR WAY

STRONG ENOUGH TO FIGHT AND LEARN

THAT RESPECT IS SOMETHING THAT YOU
EARN

BELIEVE, BELIEVE, BELIEVE, BELIEVE ME

<u>MAY 2002</u>

WITH ANGER COMES HOPE

Heart That Hangs

He was there for five days
He altered his faith
He raised his voice
He expressed his choice

He hadn't changed
His ears inflamed
The same book was still open
Read the words, you have spoken

He'd been there
With his hands
That caressed her
Heart that hangs

He had rivers of meditation
His coat of dust was a revelation
He stood there, his life sped by
Does she care? You ask why

Search for something familiar
Try to relate, but don't touch her
She will wash all of the places
She has been so there are no traces

He'd been there
With his hands
That caressed her
Heart that hangs

February 2006

Helen Care

THE BATH IN THE LOUNGE

COMING DOWN THE STAIRS

THE COLOUR BLUE IN MY HAIR

FURTHER DOWN, DOWN, DOWN

THE AURE OF THE ROOM SURROUNDS

THE SINK, CHAIRS AND BATH

THE T.V., WHICH YOU STARE AT

THERE YOU SIT SO PROUD

LAUGHING AT THE BATH IN THE LOUNGE

DECIDE TO HAVE A WASH

AND CLEAN MY HAIR

I JUMP ONTO THE BATH

ONLY TO FIND SOMEONE

ALREADY IN THERE !!!

Why the bath?

WITH ANGER COMES HOPE

Why the stairs?

Why the chairs?

Why the bath?

The bath in the lounge !!!

TRYING TO UNDERSTAND

AS BUBBLES FLOAT ON MY HAND

END WHAT HAD BEGUN

THE AURE OF THE ROOM HAS GONE

<u>1998 / 2003</u>

Helen Care

UNFULFILLED

TAKE MY HAND
WILL YOU BE THERE?
TAKE THE STAND
WILL YOU BE FAIR?

I'M DROWNING
WILL YOU SWIM
IN AFTER ME?
I NEED TO THINK

I'M FALLING
TRY AND CATCH ME
THE GROUND IS NEAR
WAITING WILL YOU BE?

I'M CRYING
WILL YOU HELP ME?
CATCH MY TEARS
FOR I CAN'T SEE

HURTING, DISTRESSED
CAN'T YOU SEE I'M IN A MESS?
FLASHBACKS MAKE ME DIGRESS
FRAGILE, I MUST CONFESS

NEVER TAUGHT THE SKILLS
TO MAKE ME SO FILLED
WITH CONFIDENCE AND HOPE
HERE I AM, UNFULFILLED

MAY 2004

WITH ANGER COMES HOPE

<u>TOMORROW</u>

Tomorrow is a long way off

I don't want to think about it

For today was bad enough

Without you adding to it

I think I've fallen off my rock

The waves are coming in fast

All on my own with my lot

Can't get enough, will it last?

In my cocoon, no butterfly

I want to feel safe and sound

Tell me the truth, no lies

You're running me out of town

In a new place, start again

Forget the past, look ahead

Helen Care

No sun here, just pouring rain

Up on the stage, boards to tread

Back to square one, oh no

Will I ever learn from this?

Slow to respond heaven knows

I need you like you need a fish

Tomorrow is a long way off

I don't want to think about it

For today is bad enough

Please don't add to this

<u>MAY 2003</u>

WITH ANGER COMES HOPE

<u>YELLOW RIBBON</u>

YELLOW RIBBON
TWISTED TURNS
WRAPPED TIGHT
AROUND MY ARMS

NO FRILLS OR BOWS
JUST A SNATCH
GRATUITOUS SEX
I CAN NOT MATCH

YELLOW SHINES
DARKENED HEART
NUMBED SOUL
TEAR ME APART

GRIP GETS TIGHTER
MY EYES CLOSE
WITH YOU INSIDE ME
FOR NO ONE KNOWS

MY GUILTY SECRET
SCARED TO DEATH
ENDURING HORROR
NOTHING IS LEFT

TIRED OF LOVE?
I DON'T UNDERSTAND
I DID WRONG
SUBJECTED TO DEMANDS

LOST MY YOUTH

TO YOUR DESIRE
YOUR YELLOW RIBBON
NOW PUT IT IN THE FIRE

**THE DAMAGE HAS BEEN DONE
THE LEGACY WILL ROLL ON
THROUGHOUT MY LIFE
THE YELLOW RIBBON
WILL BURN A HOLE
IN MY SOUL**

<u>SEPTEMBER 2003</u>

WITH ANGER COMES HOPE

<u>*MY REALITY*</u>

Menaced by something
In the corner of my eye
Haunted by the fear that
Blows through my cries

The truth comes to me
This is my reality

For the weight
On my shoulders
Now leaves me
Feeling older

The truth comes to me
This is my reality

Building up my hopes
An explosion of fire
I've never been happier
But closer to the wire

The truth comes to me
This is my reality

Give me something
Sustainable
Reach for something
Attainable

The truth comes to me
This is my reality

Helen Care

OCTOBER 2004

WITH ANGER COMES HOPE

Life's Lessons

By this ritual, she seemed to know
That her skin would acquire a different glow
The colour of night was so artificial
That her skin would crawl at your love so cynical

For she noticed love was a mystery
She would pray, love would be her fantasy
She was kept in darkness along with all your demons
She never understood, you never provided reasons

Her desire to be good, well behaved and true
To your expectations that came right on cue
Her orientations had been experienced
Up until the moment, she felt your existence

With a simple rebellion against all the lives
That surrounded her and took her by surprise
See their forms and coloured realms so much deeper
Remotely discovered as everyone's a stranger

Sent off like a rocket with a charge of power
Shooting up into space, encouraged to empower
Understanding by those who needed guidance
Can they see the light? Do they need tolerance?

Death is always near life is always a surprise
Along your journey, you'll see how the land lies
From your childhood to your adolescence

And then adulthood, we all learn life's lessons.

February 2006

WITH ANGER COMES HOPE

Balance On the Fence

_The caresses of the night before were acutely
bright
Like the multicoloured flames from artful fireworks
that came
With bursts of exploded suns and neon within the
guns
Flying comets aimed so high, they flew up so far in
the sky_

**Look at the centres of delight, shooting stars –
a piercing sight
Stand under the showers of sparks that'll save
you from the dark
She saw two scenes before her eyes, one of
death he's not alive
An image of intolerable pain, don't want to be
here again**

_The second was one of anger, so close to his
chest he asked her
To stop bringing out the worst in him as he thinks
he'll burst_
**Before the night turns to dawn, his anxiety has
now been born
He continues to lie in silence not ready to
balance on the fence**

_He gradually slides out of bed being careful not to
bang his head
His clothes slipped in his hands, getting up was so
unplanned_

He can feel her body tense, she couldn't bear the
suspense
Walking barefoot down the stairs carrying her
shoes with care

She feels so utterly weak the steps start to
creak
Finally, she reached the door, she won't see
him anymore
Her heart was paralysed from all of his hurtful
lies
Facing up to her terror and guilt, regret stops
her being still

Is it the end of the world? Will my death be
unfurled?
In a moment of passion, like it's going out of
fashion
Before the night turns to dawn, his anxiety has
now been born
He continues to lie in silence not ready to
balance on the fence

February 2006

WITH ANGER COMES HOPE

THE ISLAND MAN

YOU DON'T LOVE ME, YOU DON'T EMBRACE
ME
SO KISS ME ON THE LIPS AND THEN I'LL
FORGIVE

The music, the trees, the sounds, the leaves

THE DRUMS OF THE ISLAND WHERE YOU DID
DRUM
ONLY SOUGHT TO POSSESS THE POWER NO
LESS, YES...

Offer your body to be free, tropical winds will
begin...

TO FEEL THE PRESSURE OF FINDING THE
TREASURE
WHEN YOU SWIM GET OUT YOUR FIN

She savoured on his lips
The island's spices he sipped
He learned this was the way
To caress her and feel okay

YOU DON'T WANT TO HARM OR RAISE THE
ALARM
SO YOU'LL DEAL WITH HER GUILT THAT SHE
HAS SLOWLY BUILT

Over time, see the sign of directions of
connections

155

Helen Care

A SUBTLE SHAME OF WHO'S TO BLAME
WHO DO YOU LOVE? HAVE YOU HAD
ENOUGH?

To disunite, take a bite that leaves a sour taste
every hour

She savoured on his lips
The island's spices he sipped
He learned this was the way
To caress her and feel okay
<u>FEBRUARY 2006</u>

WITH ANGER COMES HOPE

A LOST SOUL

WILDLY PSYCHOTICALLY
OUT OF CONTROL, A LOST SOUL

MANIA QUICKLY
BURNED ITSELF IN THIS HELL

EXHAUSTING EXHILARATING
DEFINITELY DISTURBINGLY

OVER THE TOP FALLING OUT
OF MY LIFE AND MY MIND

CLEAR AS CRYSTAL
SO TORTUOUS SO VIRTUOUS

READ THE SAME PASSAGE OVER
ONLY TO REALISE IT'S FULL OF LIES

NO MEMORY NO CAPACITY
TO REMEMBER SO FORGET HER

I WOULD STARE OUT THE WINDOW
WITH NO IDEA OF MY FEAR

FOR MY MIND IS MY FRIEND
ENDLESS WORDS GO UNHEARD

SUCH LAUGHTER RESCUED ME
FROM THE PAINFUL AND UNFORGIVABLE

SUCH LOYALTY WAS WASTED

Helen Care

TURNED ON ME SO FEROCIOUSLY

**WILDLY PSYCHOTICALLY
OUT OF CONTROL, A LOST SOUL**

<u>NOVEMBER 2006</u>

WITH ANGER COMES HOPE

Twist and Turn

Life is not enough

When you can't call

Your soul your own

So I continually fall

Over and over and over again

Is it me or am I going insane?

Feeling at a loss in all this confusion

Compounded by thoughts of intrusion

That twists and turns inside my head

Leaving me isolated by what you said

I really can't take much more you know

I need to escape, leaving friends and foes

I've lost the light at the end of my tunnel

What do I do to stop this tossing and tumble?

Helen Care

When I need to relax and get some sleep

For nightmares, flashbacks and secrets I keep

Life is not enough

When you can't call

Your soul your own

So I continually fall

<u>February 2004</u>

Such a Bore

Handle the journey
Into a world
With the knowledge
Beauty unfurls

Skills to navigate
To be solvent
A limited approach
Came and went

**Consisting almost
Entirely of chores
Rigid cocoons
Such a bore**

Cross the street
Try to avoid
A dark world
So annoyed

Really surprising
Flee the scary
Empty feelings
That becomes reality

**Consisting almost
Entirely of chores
Rigid cocoons
Such a bore**

February 2005

Helen Care

YOU KEPT ON

**You kept on kissing my feet placed in isolation
we meet
Call on the bird of paradise I can't stop this
mad life**

I can shop for nothing why not I think I'm mad
We don't use these words that make us feel so
sad

Banish the word of lunatic, the asylum no longer
works
Insanity comes to us all where oppression we all
have heard

We distance our oppression but still remain
neglected
We live in the shadow so precarious and dejected

Catapulted into melodrama frightened of losing
control
We don't understand madness we understand
little of our role

For the ordeal of insanity and the struggle of
human spirit
To rise above and control the feeling of being 'with
it'

Insanity happens to other people brushing their
wings with madness

WITH ANGER COMES HOPE

For we can choose to hide or face up to our
shame and distress

We can learn from our condition of birth, death
and love
Where hate, passion and denial prove to be far
too much

You sometimes behave erratically; you may think
the world is against you
From passiveness to aggressive, my madness for
you is a clue

You kept on kissing my feet placed in isolation
we meet
Call on the bird of paradise I can't stop this
mad life

MAY 2006

163

Helen Care

She Smiled As She Smirked

She always wanted
To know how things worked
Why do stairs stand up?
She smiled as she smirked

Why do things stand up?
Why do things fall down?
Make up a story as to why
An understanding to astound

Suffered for not knowing
The difference of before
And after, but because
Of two destinies' I'm sure

She had many characteristics
She could always amuse herself
Even in times of solitude
Without having to rely on anyone else

She got used to going to churches
She'd turn and say "Shall we go in?"
Later she rebelled saying that
She couldn't bear such a sin

Watching ghastly cartoons on TV
Becoming more demanding
For God knows what I remember
But I forget your understanding

You can bend wood if you steam it

WITH ANGER COMES HOPE

The kitchen is a cottage industry
On such an extraordinary adventure
That all works out for society

She always wanted
To know how things worked
Why do the stairs stand up?
She smiled as she smirked

February 2005

Helen Care

WORDS OF COMFORT

MANICALLY EUPHORIC
LIGHTEN THE ATMOSPHERE
JUMP OUT THE WINDOW
TRY NOT TO LIVE IN FEAR

PROTECT ME FROM REGISTERING
WHAT HAPPENED TO MY MIND
SOMETIMES IT IS FRIGHTENING
IT'S HARD TO CONTROL I FIND

LEAPING OUT OF A CAR
ON THE DUAL CARRIAGEWAY
BUT THEN MY MOOD CHANGED
ARRIVE AT THE HEARSAY

As soon as I was through
The door that opened my heart
To listening to your words
Of comfort that will go far

I WAS SITTING ON THE EDGE
OF MY BOWING HEAD
INSIDE MYSELF I WEEP
DEFEATED MY HEART BLED

PLEASE TELL ME YOU LOVE ME
CONTINUALLY WITHOUT SPACE
TO FIND IN MY HEART
EMOTIONS YOU CAN'T BACKDATE

OBSESSED WITH FINDING OUT

WITH ANGER COMES HOPE

**OF WHAT I CAN'T UNDERSTAND
IT'S ALL A TRAGEDY TO ME
I NEED TO KEEP MY HAND**

*As soon as I was through
The door that opened my heart
To listening to your words
Of comfort that will go far*

JANUARY 2005

The Colour Is You

At first like small children's steps
Running through tall dry rushes next
Then heavier strides on hollow wood
Sharp on the outside soft like she could…

Tap the drum skins thumped and slapped
She wants to win, her smile collapsed
Her bones showed up in the glistening sea
So wild and rough leaping so quickly

In emerald green
And indigo blue
Orange tangerine
The colour is you

Colours of fruit the scent of flowers
Are not a fluke, they last for hours
There were places where the beat
Of blood embraces her body complete…

With separation from the speed
Of her isolation that runs deep
Her voice so rich she sang with joy
The notes she hit, love she did employ

In emerald green
And indigo blue
Orange tangerine
The colour is you

February 2006

168

WITH ANGER COMES HOPE

<u>Soft and Bright</u>

Among the dark face there was a pale one
Shell-white in places that smiles like she's done
Leaving her hair black so it won't reflect
Depth so matter of fact will she ever detect…

**His head's so round, his brow's so wide
Cheeks so full of sound, his eyes soft and
bright**

Her fingers on the drum so nimble with vengeance
Rippling hips that'd begun to tear down her
defence
Swimming in the sea showing off her bones
That climbs the trees before she has flown… as…

**His head's so round, his brow's so wide
Cheeks so full of sound, his eyes soft and
bright**

Her muscles are strong but invisible like a cat
Whose tail is so long it doesn't know where it's at
The diffusion of colour gave her a gesture
So nervous of splendour, this moment she'll
treasure

**His head's so round, his brow's so wide
Cheeks so full of sound, his eyes soft and
bright**

The softness of the wind flows down to the warm
sea

Helen Care

Where it exploded behind in cycles all around me
They say life is sweet but when you stop playing
Our broken hearts will meet, then you'll catch me
swaying…as...

**His head's so round, his brow's so wide
Cheeks so full of sound, his eyes soft and
bright**

<u>February 2006</u>

WITH ANGER COMES HOPE

DAWNING

SHE WATCHED HIM CLOSE THE WINDOW
LIGHT THE LAMP THAT GAVE A GLOW
HE OPENED THE DOOR THAT LED TO THE
PORCH
AND INTO THE WARMTH, HOPE HAS BEEN
CAUGHT

HE HAD A GENTLENESS THAT ENCOURAGED
PEACE
FOR HER BODY AND SOUL JUMPED WITH A
LEAP
HIS IMAGE IS CRACKING WITH HIS RESTLESS
BONES
LOST IN THE MIDST, PLEASE TAKE ME HOME

YOU ARRIVE CHARGED AND ELECTRIFIED
WITH SUCH DELIGHT HER HEART'S ON FIRE
THE HONEY FLOWS LIKE THE BEE
WHO THEN STINGS AND THEN FLEES

ALL YOUR DESIRES WAFTED ON THE SHORE
FROM THE WAVES THAT EBB AND FLOW
ONCE MORE
LIKE THE SENSUAL TIDE THAT COVERS
YOUR DESIRE
WITH EVERY LAPPING WAVE THAT GETS
HIGHER AND HIGHER

LIKE AN UNREACHABLE DANCE DRESSED
UP WITH COLOUR

Helen Care

UNPARALLELED IN SPLENDOUR IN
RELATION TO EACH OTHER
SHE WISHES HE WAS THERE SO CLOSE AND
SO NEAR
SHE SAYS SHE CAN'T WAIT, LONELINESS
SHE WILL FEAR

HE'S BENDING TOWARDS HER LIKE A TREE
OF FAITHFULNESS
WHISPERING TO HER DREAM HE FINDS HER
WITH A COMPASS
THE MIRAGES FLOW, ENDLESSLY ALLURING
INTO THE NIGHT GLOW THAT IS DAWNING

FEBRUARY 2006

WITH ANGER COMES HOPE

<u>One Person's Madness</u>

Destroy the many foundations
That underlies your sinking
There is no clear boundary
Between your sanity and my thinking

A boundary between normal and ill
For are they discrete and distinct?
Can we forgive the many fantasies?
And ailments forged by the shrink?

From basic assumptions to genetic causes
Their needs for far more explanations
Madness is not something you choose
For we all run this risk of these damnations

Are there many symptoms in common
So that's impossible to tell them apart
You can't put people in pigeonholes
Just to make it a more comfortable art!

Is it a meaningful way of coping?
To breakdown and lose your defences
Chemical strait jackets and pills
Wear you down and stifle your senses

Am I the only one that's mad?
For it can happen to anyone
One person's madness is another's sanity
From being brave to becoming numb!!!

<u>February 2004</u>

173

Helen Care

So Why Do We Pretend?

It's terrifying that
So many nations
Can be drawn into
Such abominations

Such excuses for war
While we sit by
Watching civilisations
Get abused and slowly die

The abuse of a nation
That will turn round and bite
So out of sight
It's just not right

So harsh and so cruel
Weapons of mass destruction
What about sanctions?
Nuclear war leaves us anxious

A regime of change
With a need of less harm
Thinking it would be over
In six weeks, such alarm

Absolute lies
Absolute spin
Does it matter what side you're on?
Does it matter who will win?

A justifiable excuse

WITH ANGER COMES HOPE

Is that your defence?
A righteous war
So why do we pretend?

December 2004

Helen Care

"SALLY"

A mother who was wrongly put into jail
For killing her two sons, has died as she failed…
To recover from her conviction of an appalling
miscarriage
Of justice she suffered, leaving her with baggage

Totally discredited her conviction quashed
After studies suggested evidence was rushed
An earlier appeal failed but the case referred
For a hearing to decide, it was time she was heard

She was not victorious there are no winners
They all lost out to the powers that be sinners
Did the nightmare really end then the decision
reversed
Three years and three months in jail, that was the
worst

Given two life sentences so reviled and abused
Her inmates convinced of her innocence, so chose
To hear her husband who tirelessly campaigned
To clear his wife's name amid judgements of
shame

For she died at home, for she never recovered
She was a loving mother and wife who suffered…
This appalling tragedy leaving her only child
Motherless and alone, the family name defiled

She wanted her life back, once so happy and
content

WITH ANGER COMES HOPE

Now disgraced and lost, in turmoil not Heaven
sent
She would never be the same, her life now
tragically at an end
Ended by justice and grief, her broken heart they
couldn't mend

Sally,
Hope you found peace
From your traumatic life
So full of pain, now released.
MARCH 2007

Helen Care

SHARE LOVE AND ENJOY

I'VE REACHED THE STAGE
OF PERSONAL DEVELOPMENT
WHERE I'M ABLE TO OVERIDE
A NEGATIVE IMPEDIMENT

AFTER ALL IT'S ALWAYS
ME THAT CHOOSES
WHAT GOES ON IN MY MIND
WHAT MY SANITY LOSES

I SUSPECT IT'S COMMON
TO ME AND TO YOU
THAT WE FEEL UNCONSCIOUSLY
PUT A LID ON FEELING BLUE

THE SUFFERING ALL AROUND
THE FEAR OF LOSING FACE
BUT IT INEVITABLY FADES
TRY TO CONNECT TO THIS PLACE

THE TENDENCY TO GENERATE
AN INNATE FEAR OF WRONG
WHERE YOU LIMIT YOUR JOY
TRY TO EXPRESS IT IN A SONG

ACCENTUATE THE SUBSEQUENT
SORROW AS JOY FADES
DON'T GET YOUR MONEY'S WORTH
REGRETS COME FAR TOO LATE

FOR IT IS OUR DUTY

WITH ANGER COMES HOPE

TO BOND SORROW AND JOY
TAKE AS MUCH AS POSSIBLE
SHARE LOVE AND ENJOY

<u>FEBRUARY 2005</u>

HOPE NEVER COMES TOO LATE

I need to change it will be strange
To put my life in order and cross the border
To put my wrongs right, I won't give up the
fight
I will only win if I don't give in

Remember all the time you felt love deep
inside
You have so much to give, will my heart
forgive...
You yet again like the rain
You pour your heart out, you open up your
mouth

And start to scream, just like a bad dream
That wakes me up, I think I've had enough
Was I born to lose? Did I want to choose?
Between good and evil, life's been such an
upheaval...

Into the darker side that blew my mind
Have I gone insane? Am I to blame?
For all the hurt, that's kept me alert
And on my toes like nobody knows...

What I've been through, like you, this is
nothing new
We've all tasted loss and swallowed the cost
It's time to heal, to become more real
To grow in abundance in gaining tolerance

WITH ANGER COMES HOPE

So take your time
To cross the line
Between love and hate
Hope never comes too late

FEBRUARY 2006

Printed in the United Kingdom
by Lightning Source UK Ltd.
130050UK00001B/4-36/P

9 781847 474711